Poop Coloring Book

Something to Do While You Poo (Pocket Edition)

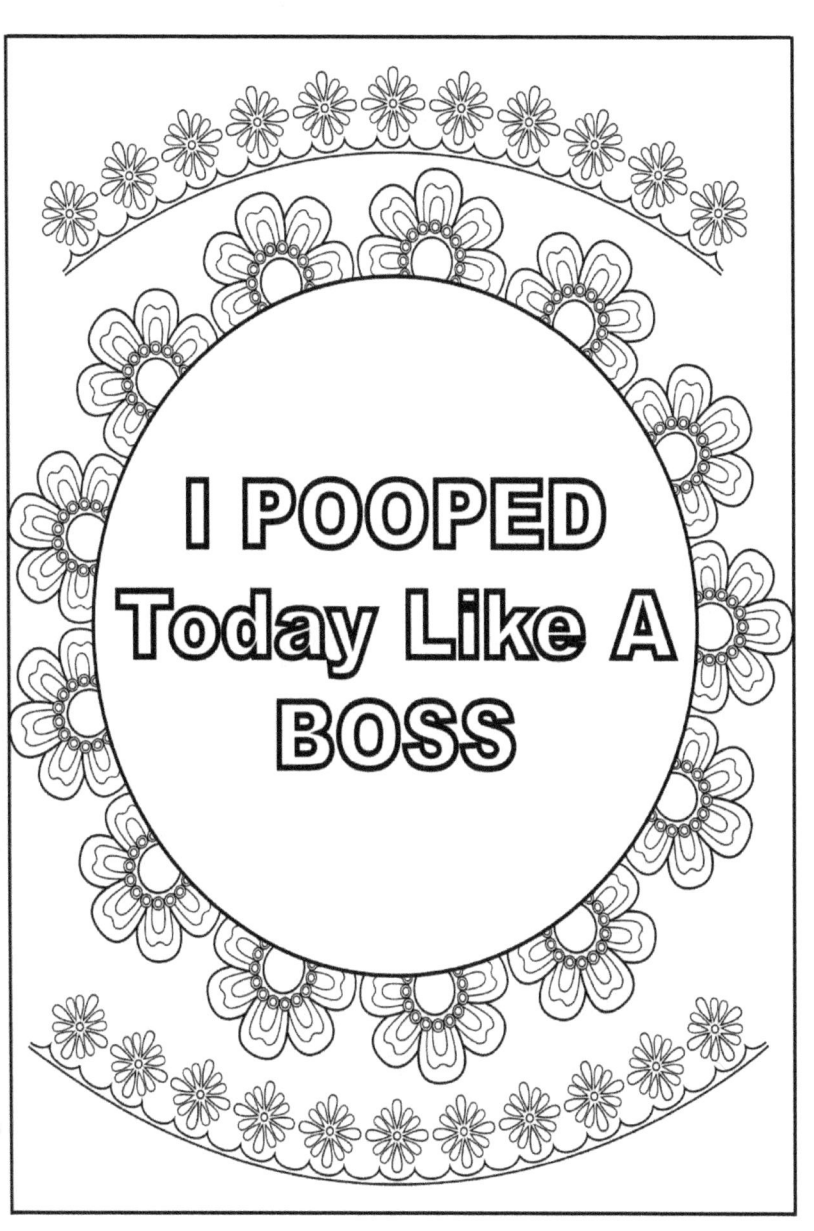

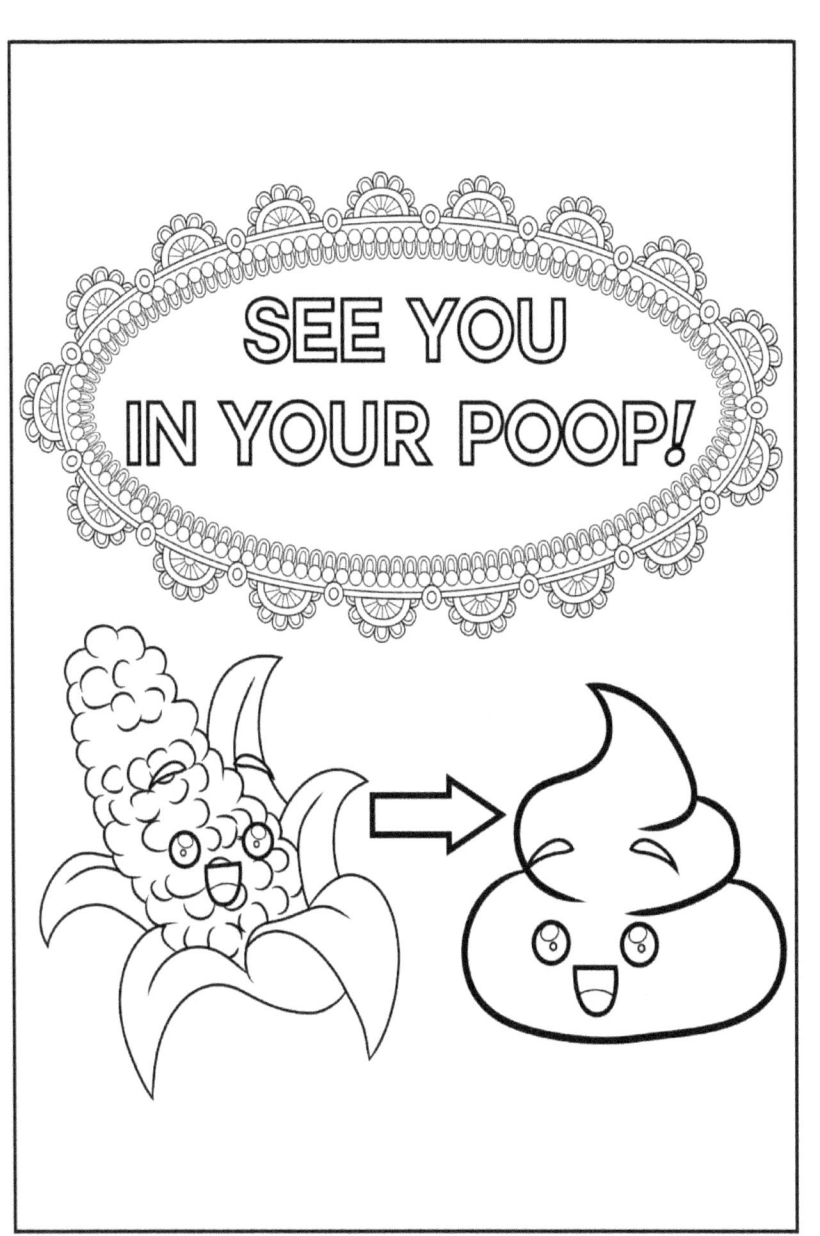

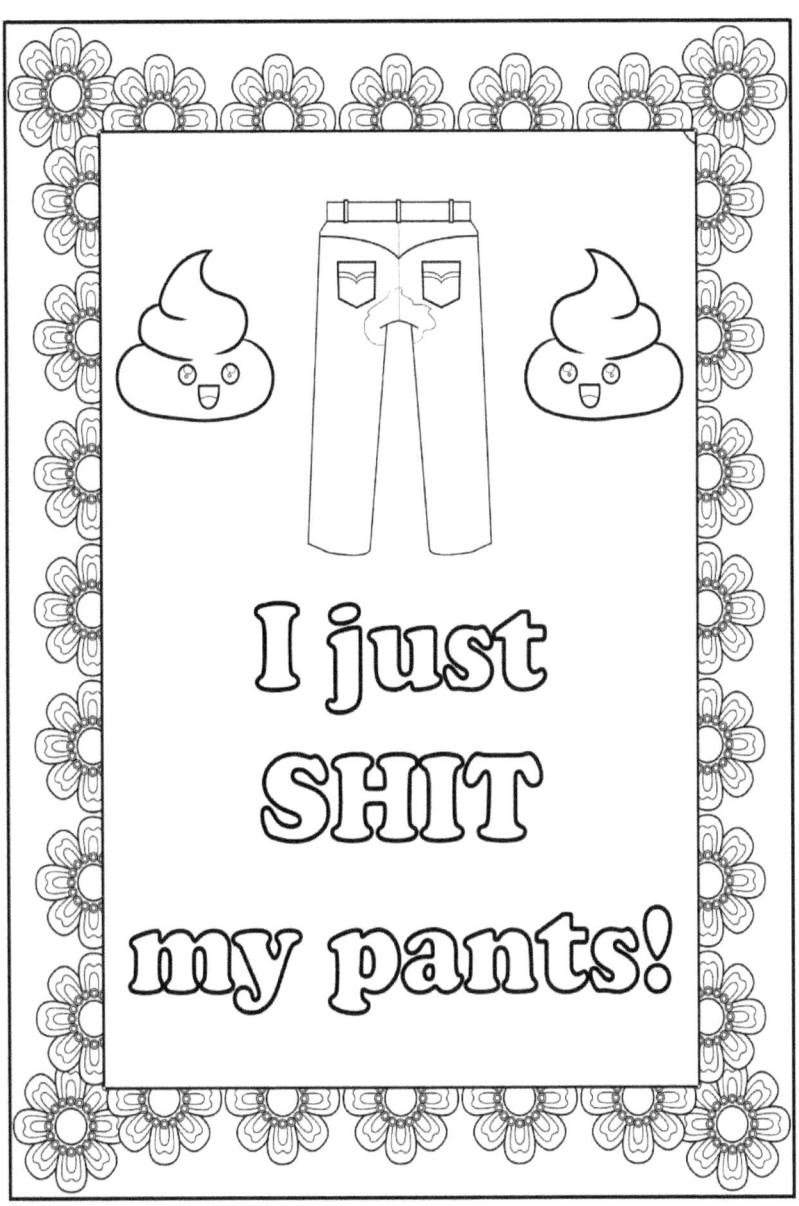

If We Hold On

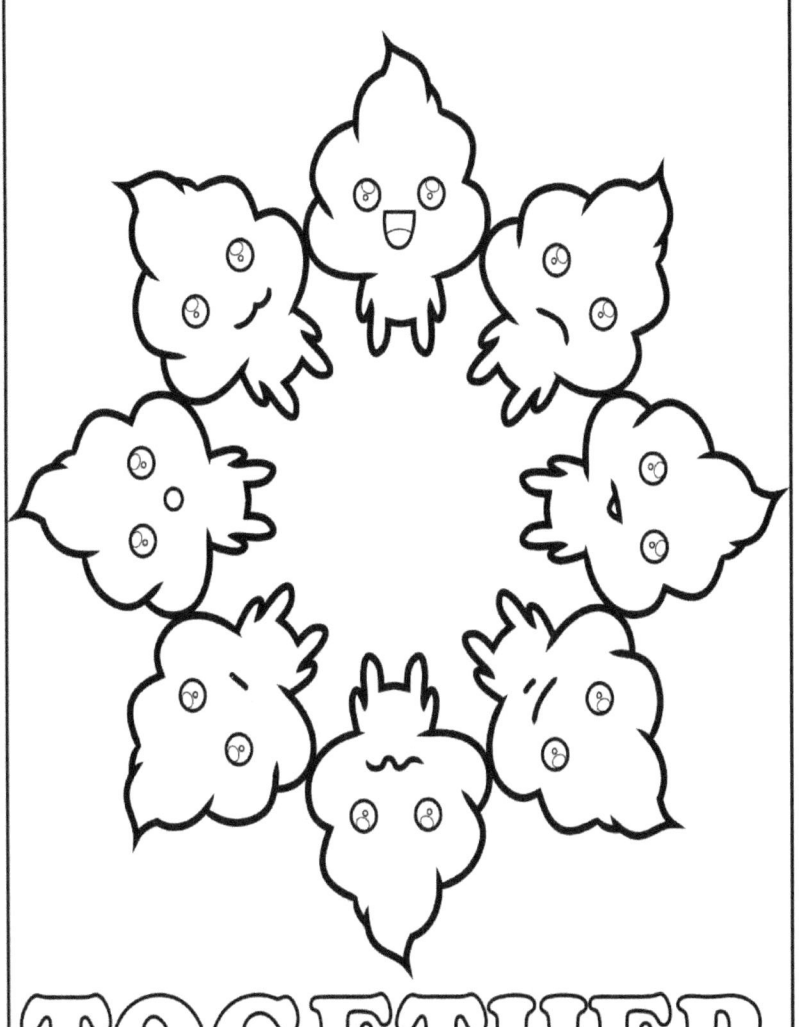

TOGETHER

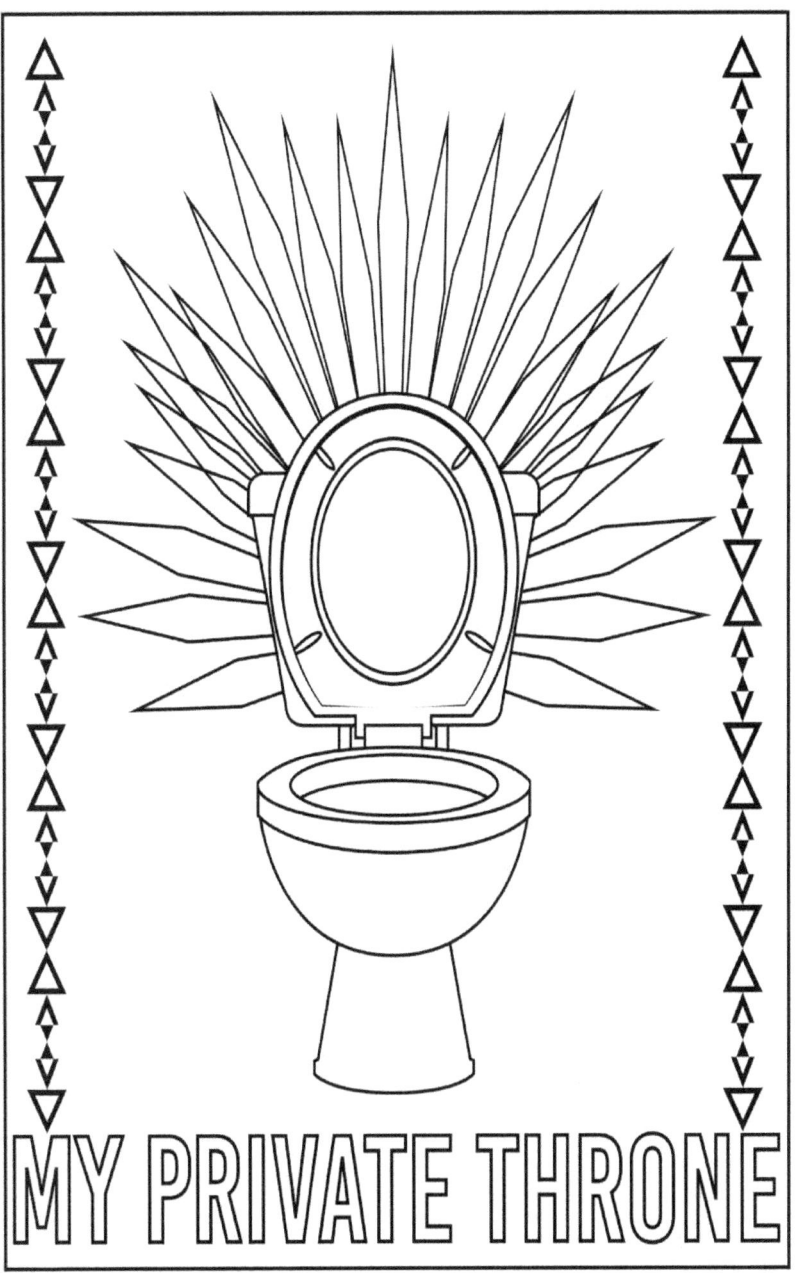

MY PRIVATE THRONE

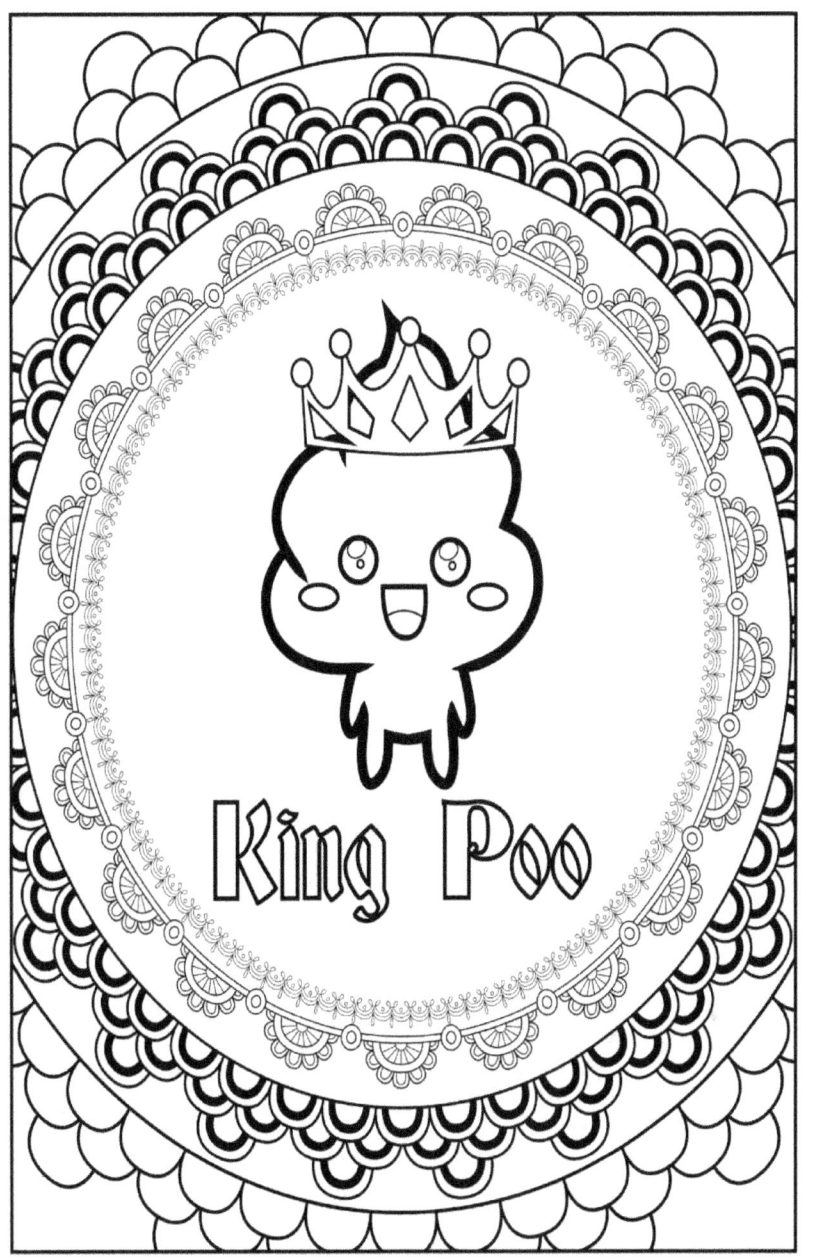

The Six Shades of Poop

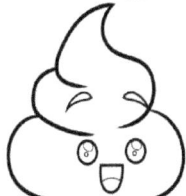

Brown: You're fine. Poop is naturally brown due to the bile produced in your liver

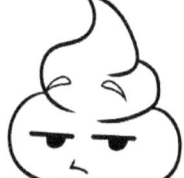

Black: It could mean that you're bleeding internally due to ulcer or cancer. Some vitamins containing iron or bismuth subsalicylate could cause black poop too. Pay attention if it's sticky, and see a doc if you're worried.

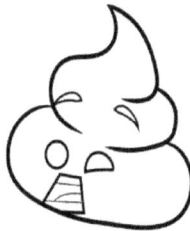

Green: Food may be movie through your large intestine too quicly. Or you could have eaten lots of green leafy veggies, or green food colouring.

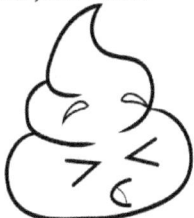

Light-coloured, white, or clay-coloured: If it's not what you're normally seeing, it could mean a bile duct obstruction. Some medscould cause this too. See a doc.

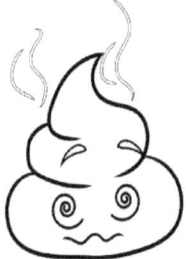

Yellow: Greasy, foul-smelling yellow poop indicates excess fat, which could be due to a malabsorption disorder like celiac disease.

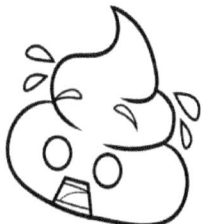

Blood-stained or Red: Blood in your poop could be a symptom of cancer. Always see a doc right away if you find blood in your stool.

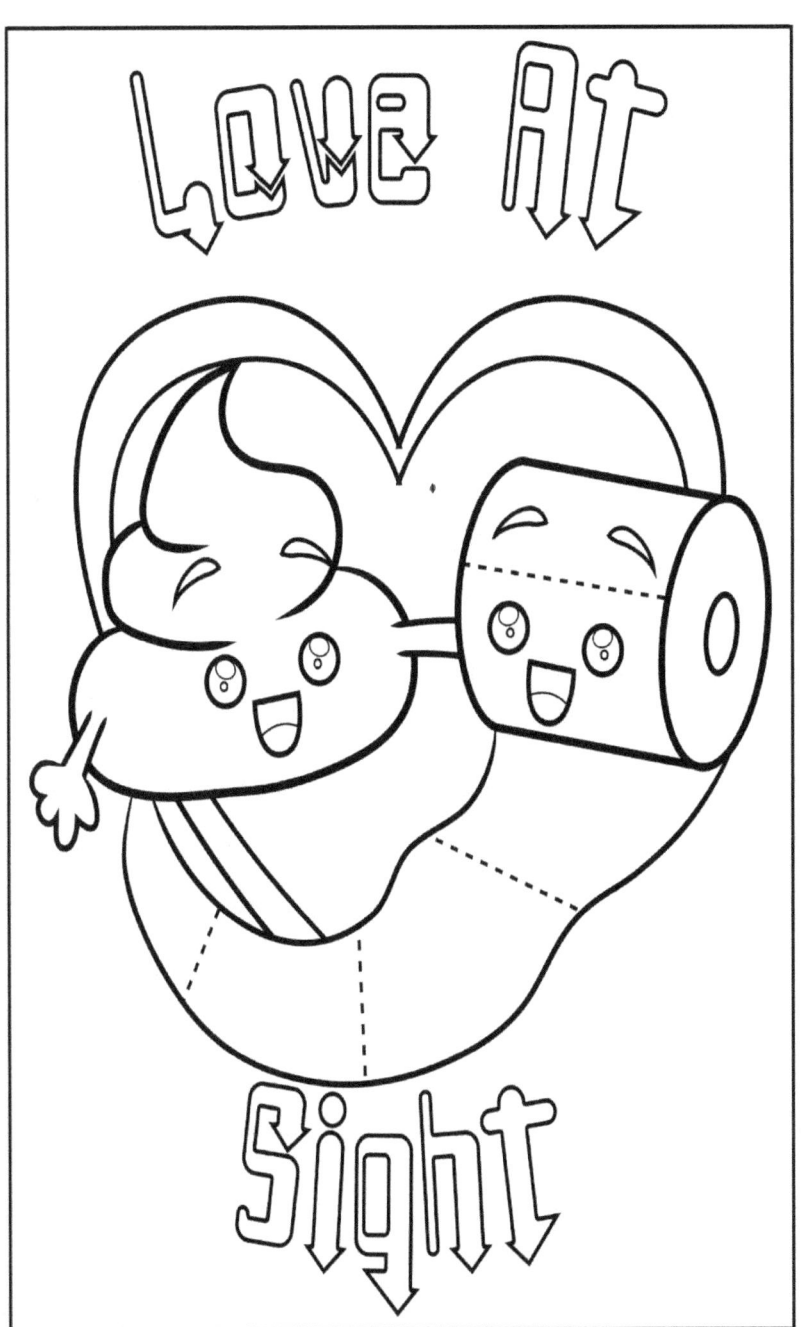

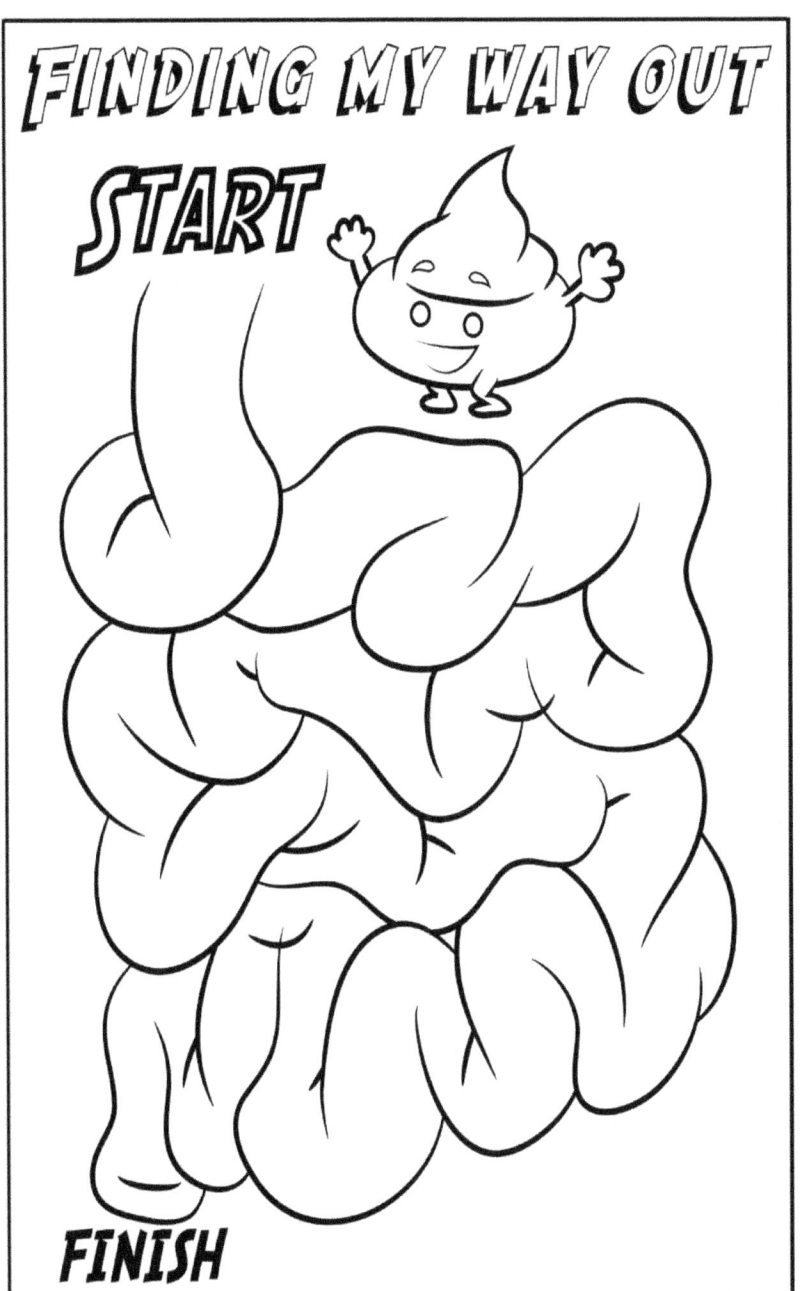

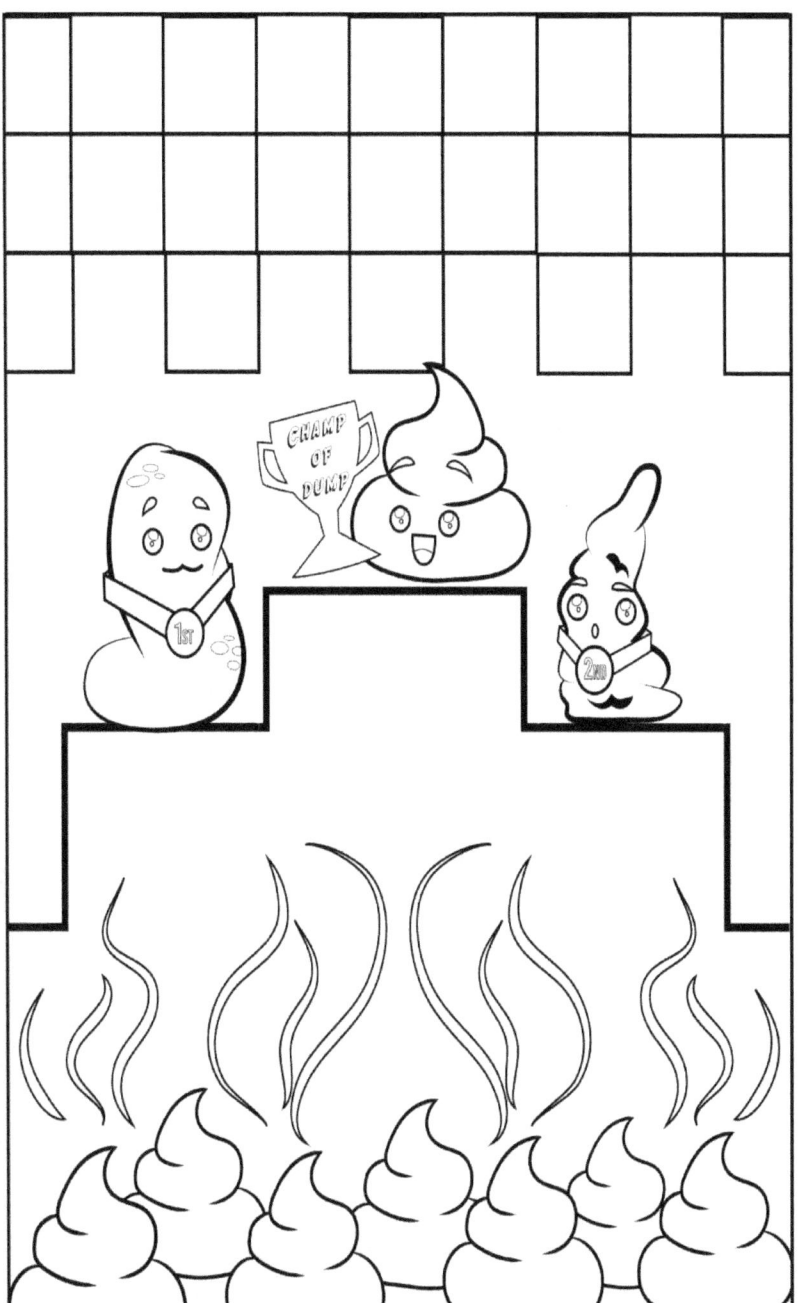

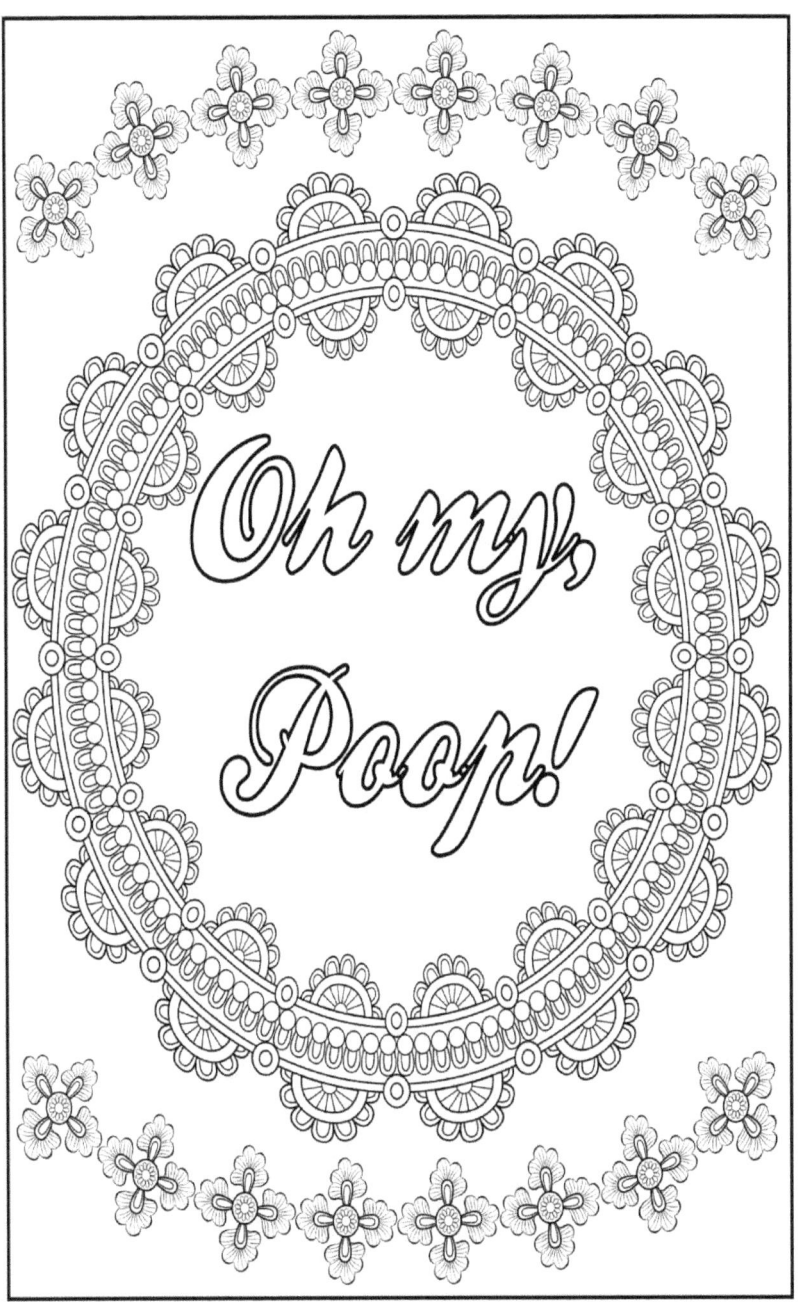

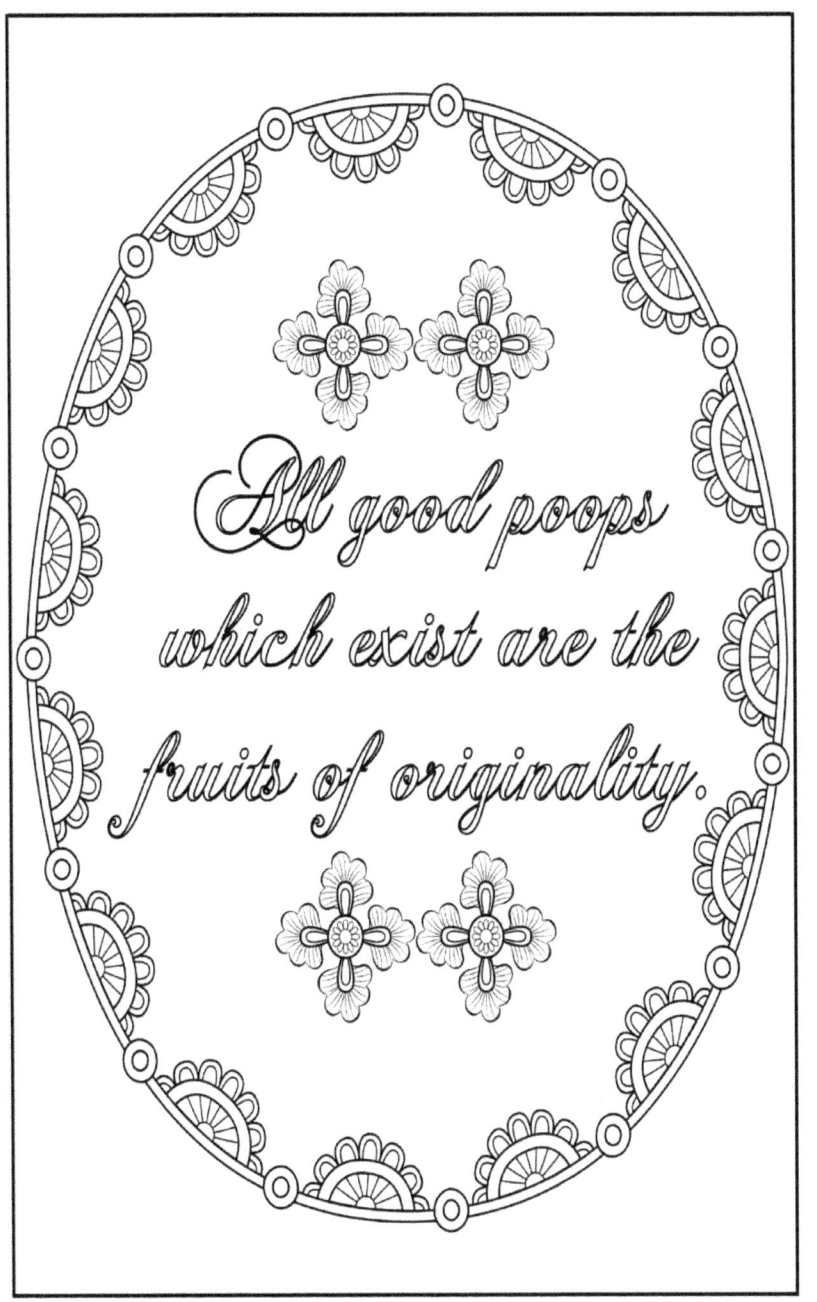

All good poops which exist are the fruits of originality.

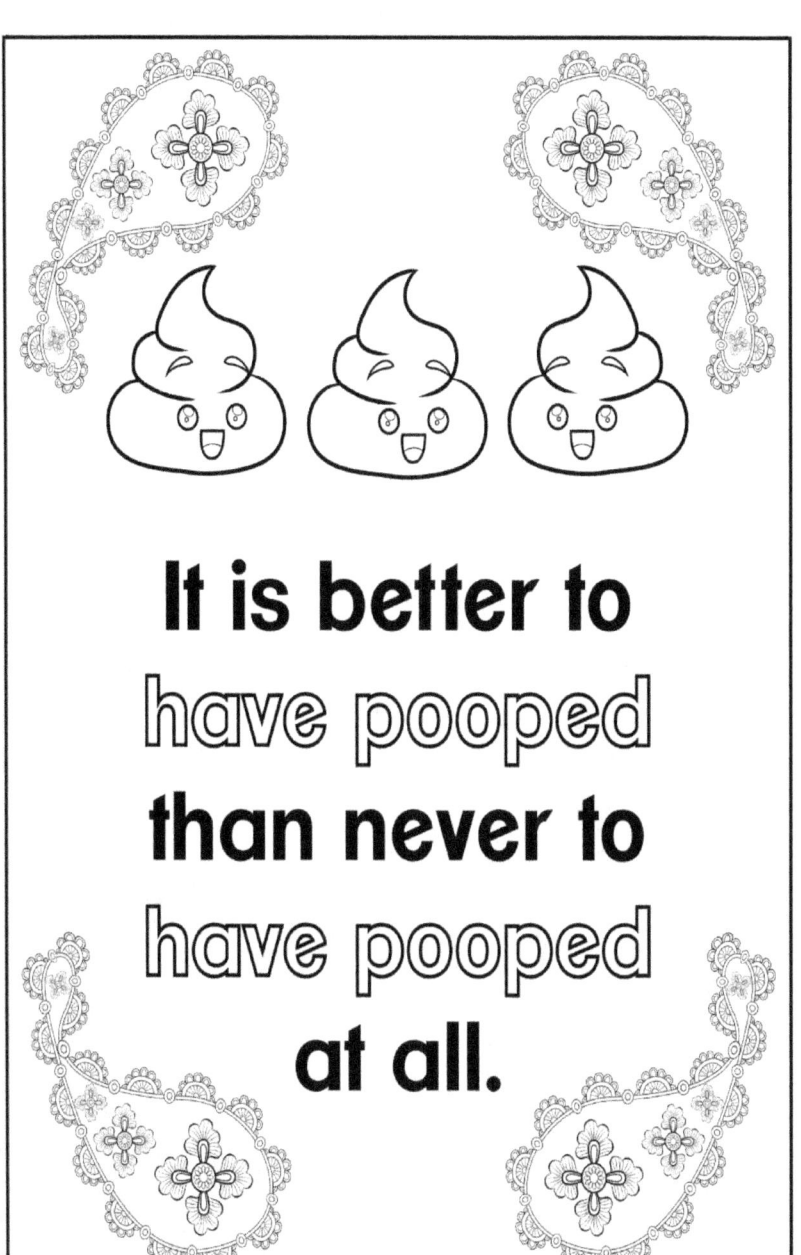

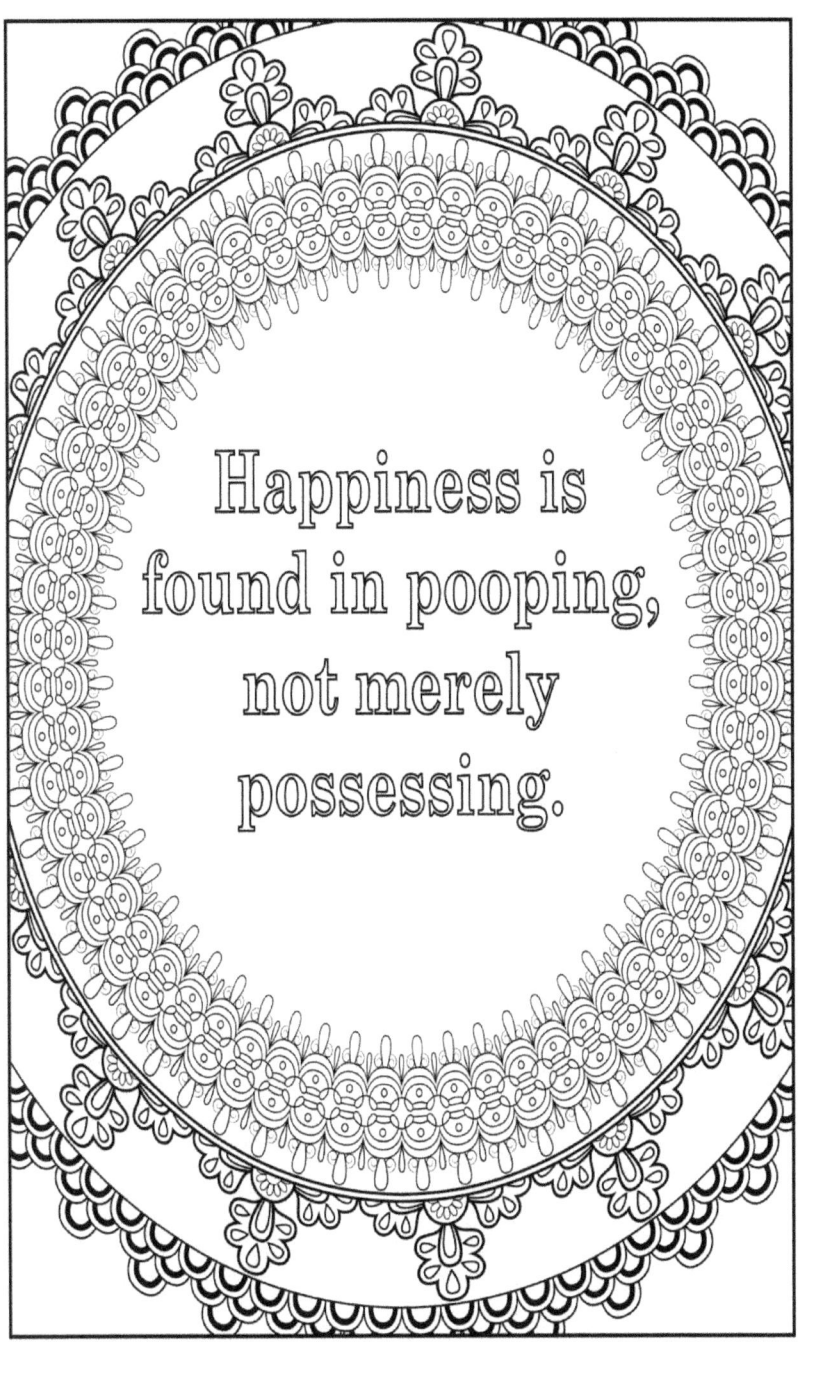

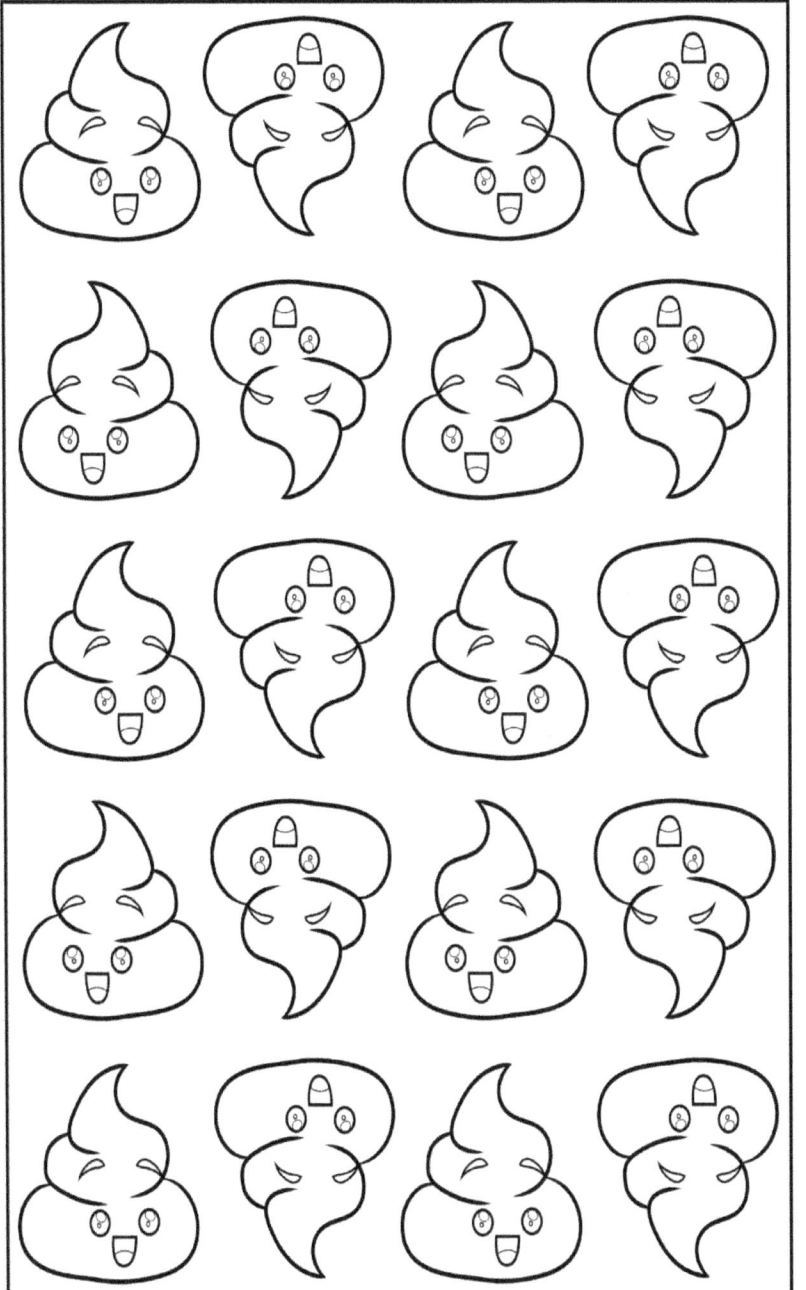

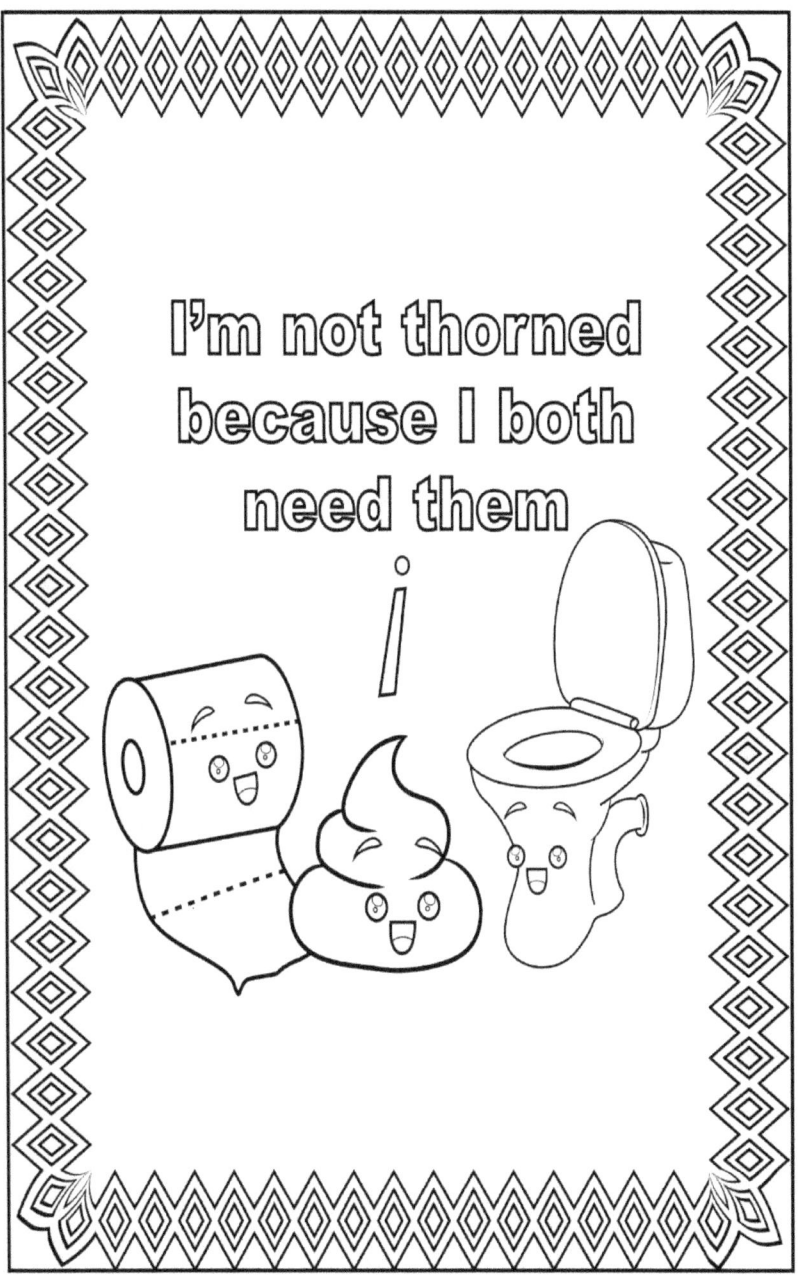

Release the

Kraken

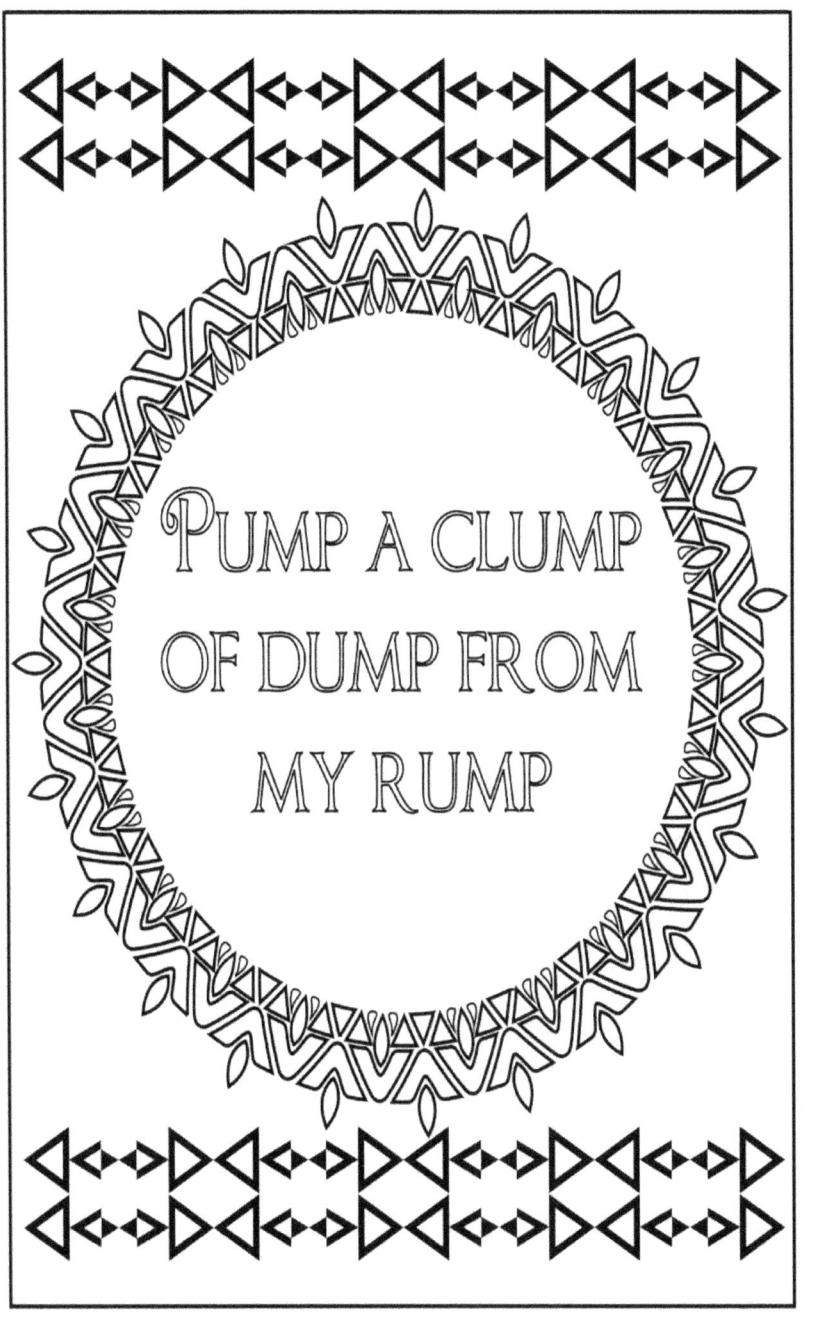

PUMP A CLUMP
OF DUMP FROM
MY RUMP

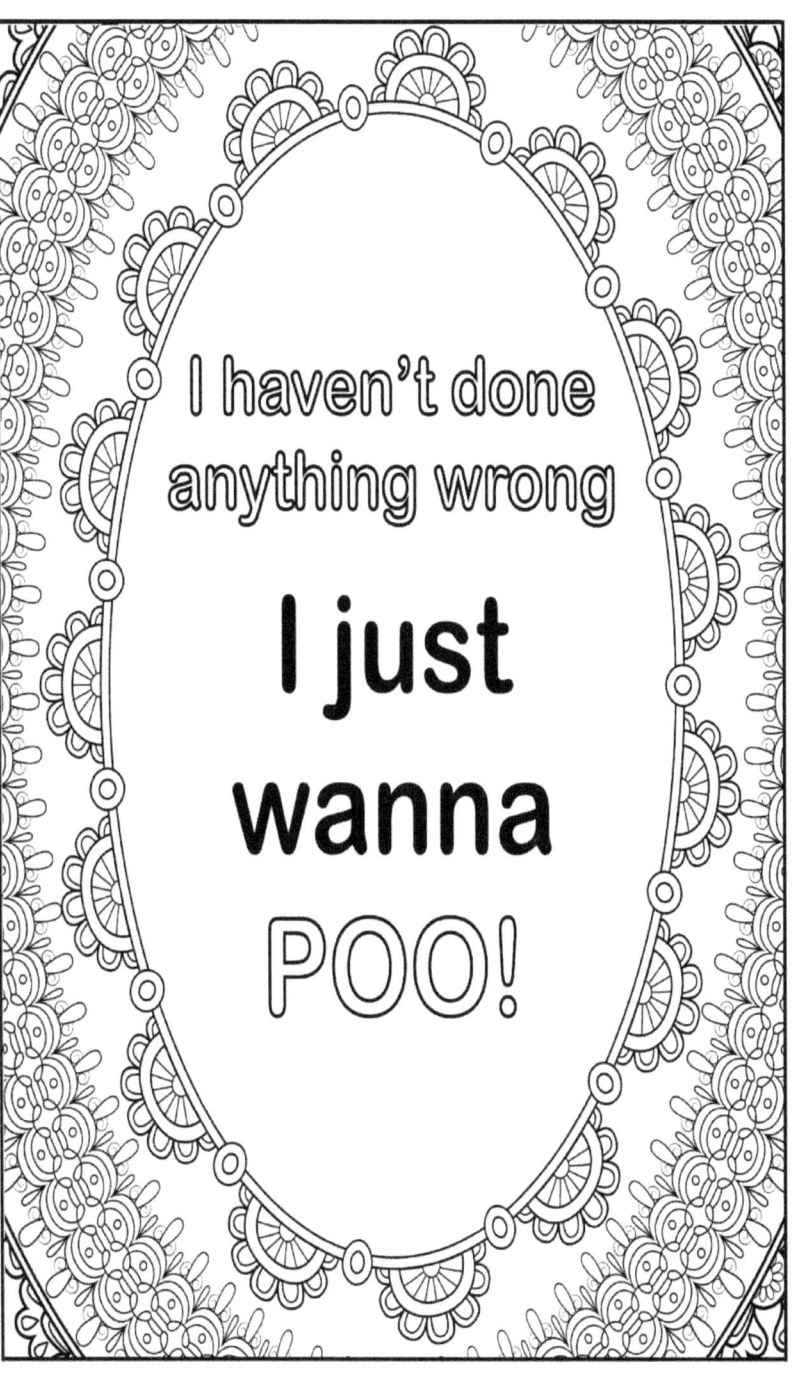

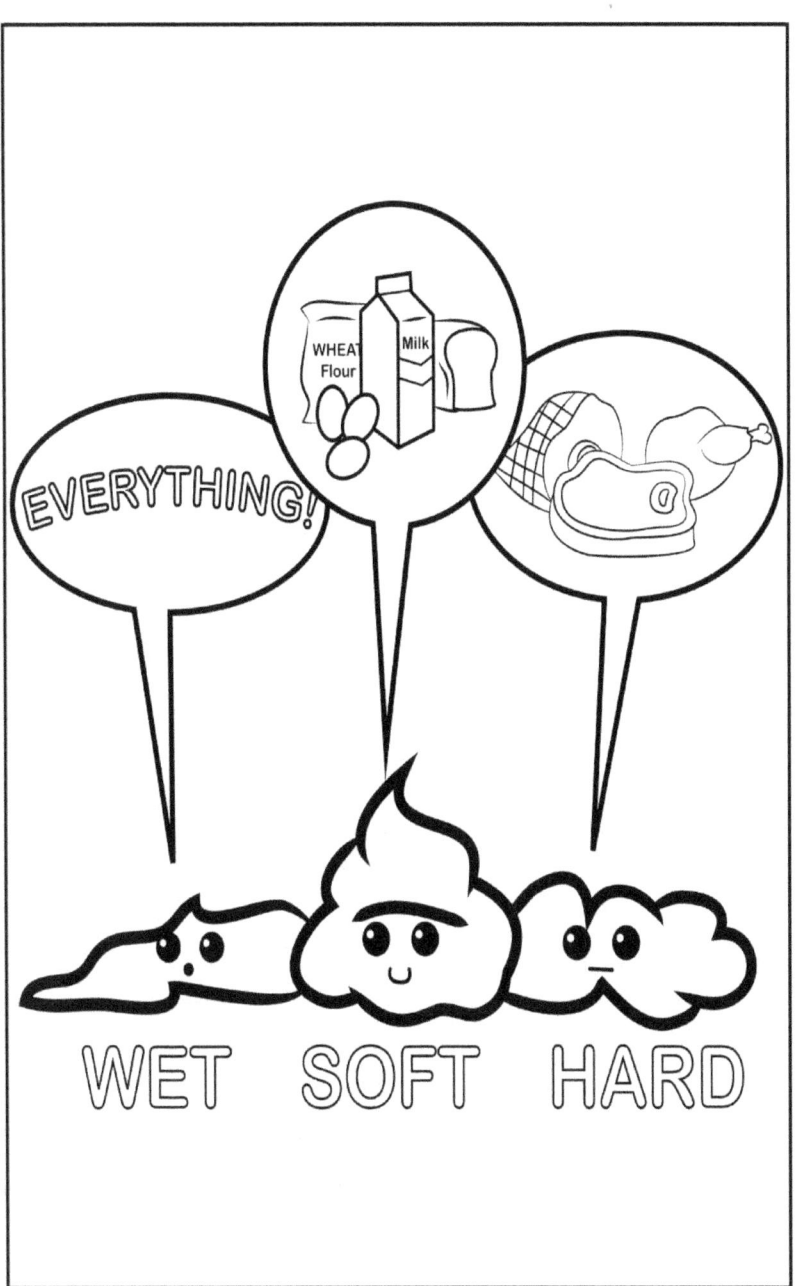

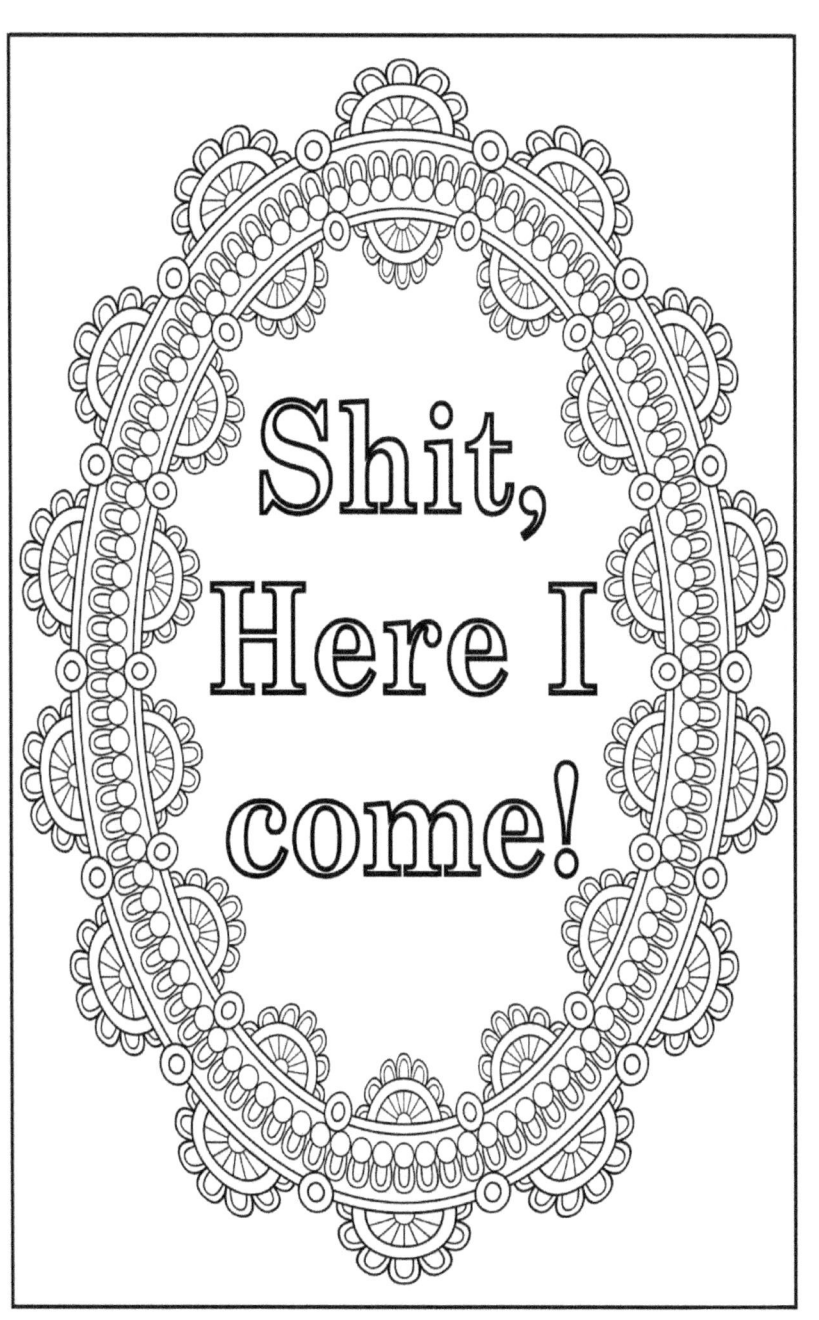

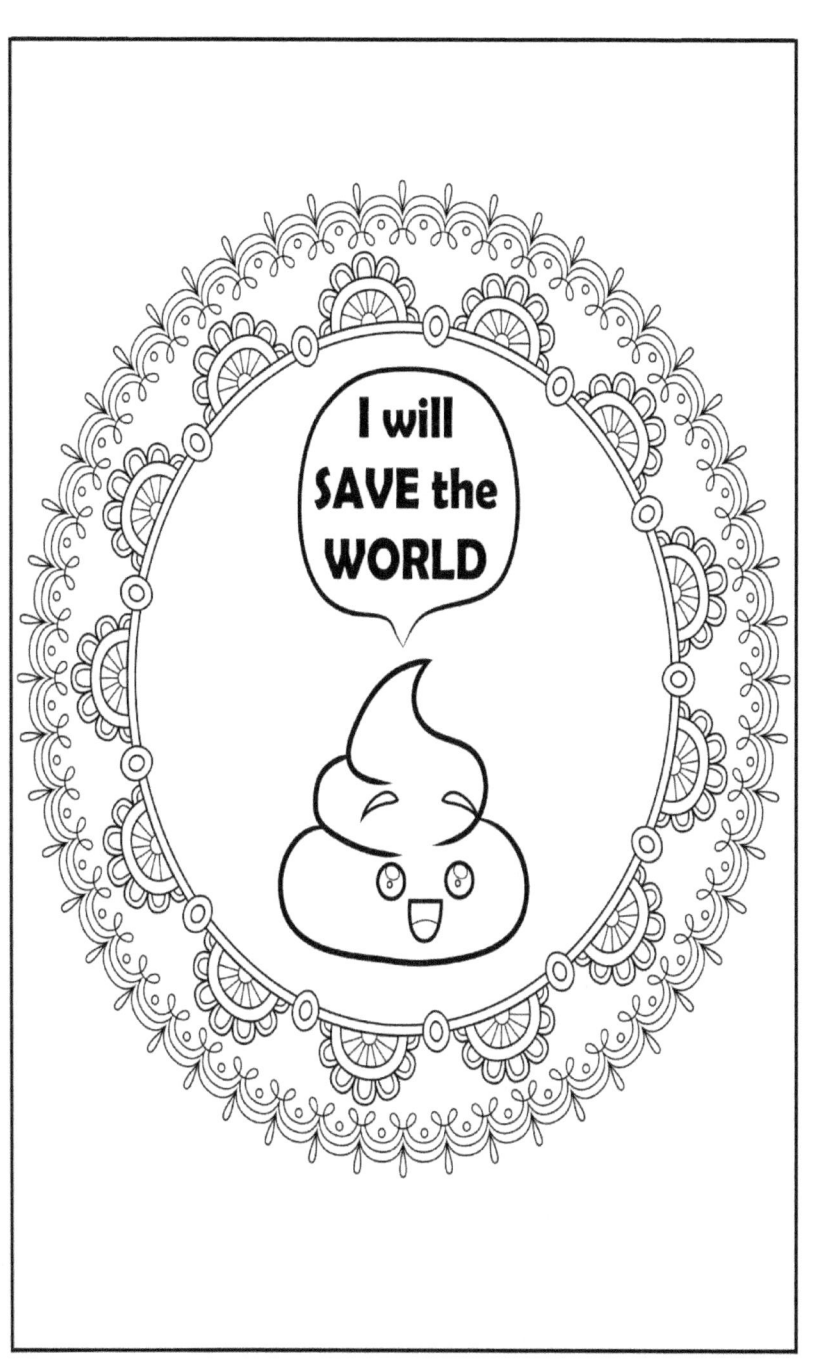

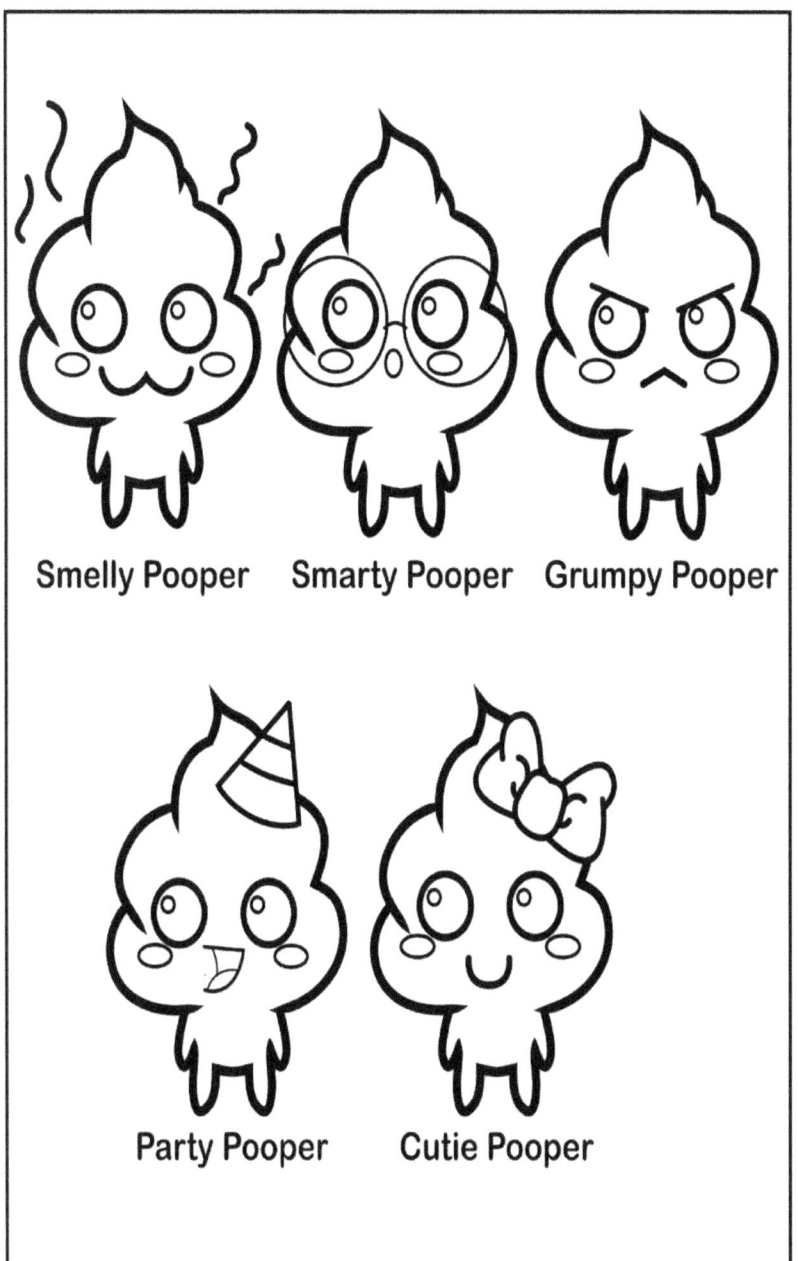

Smelly Pooper Smarty Pooper Grumpy Pooper

Party Pooper Cutie Pooper

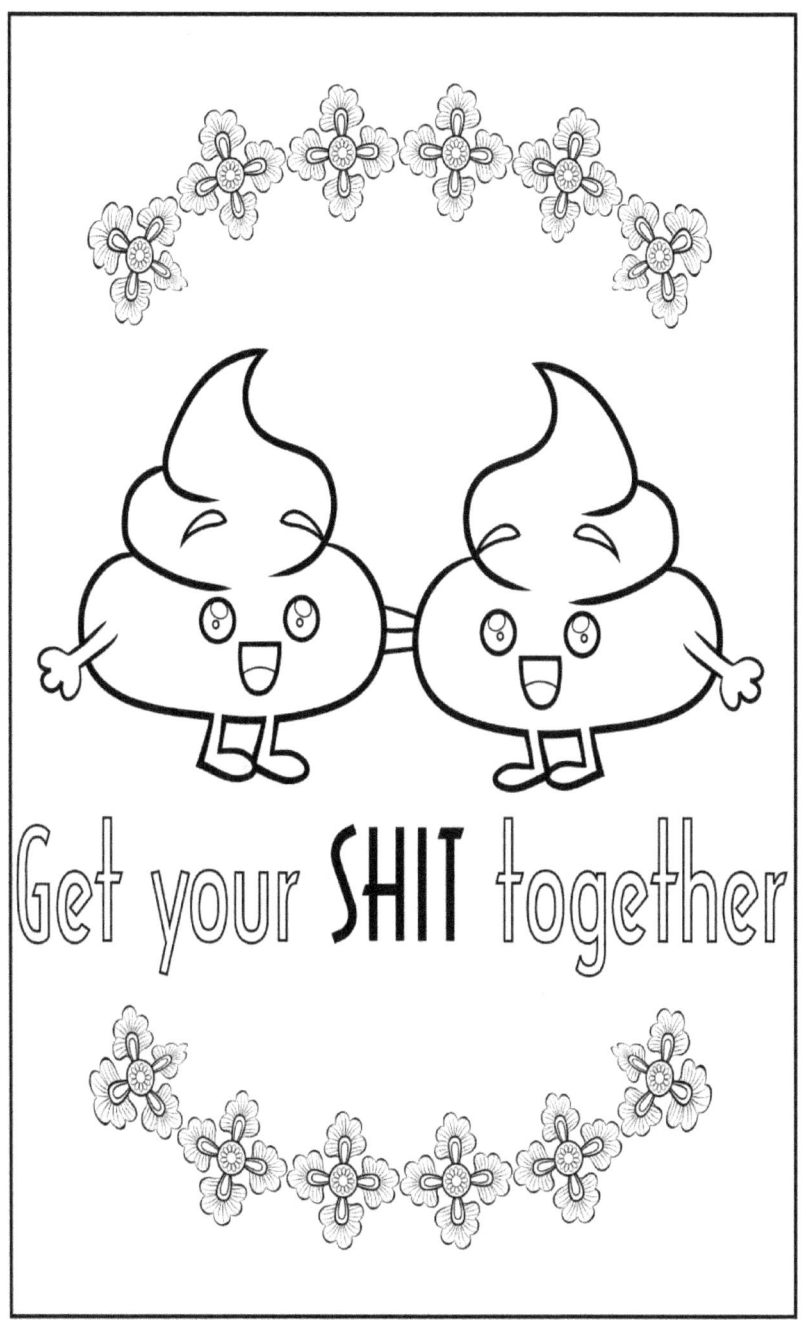

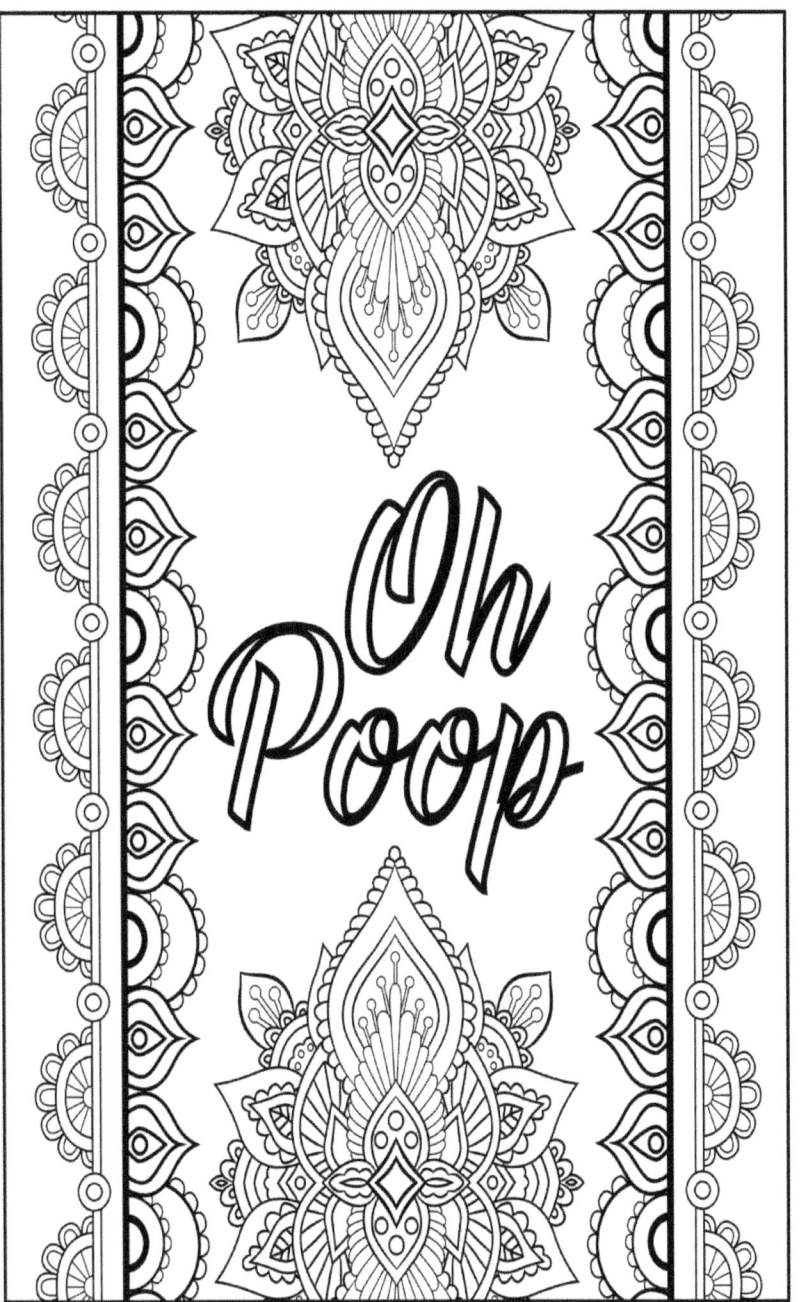

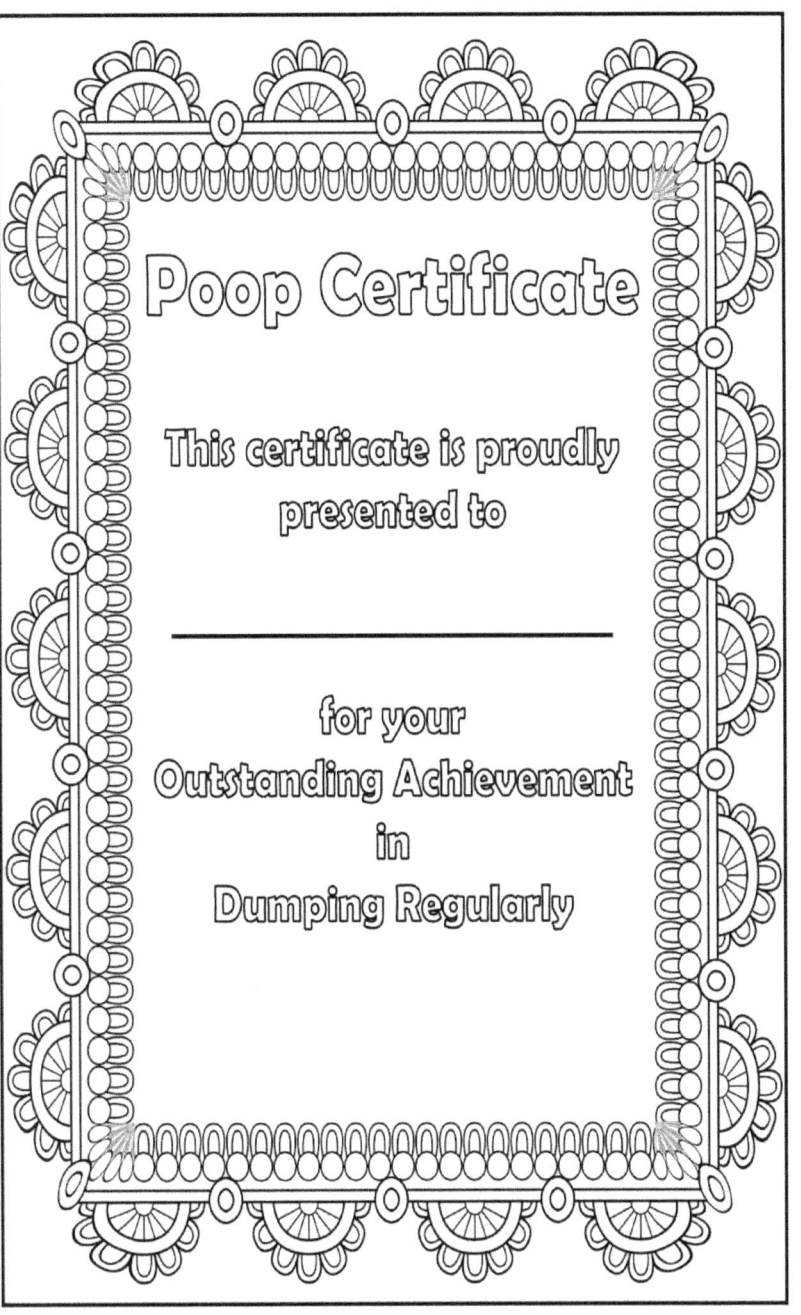

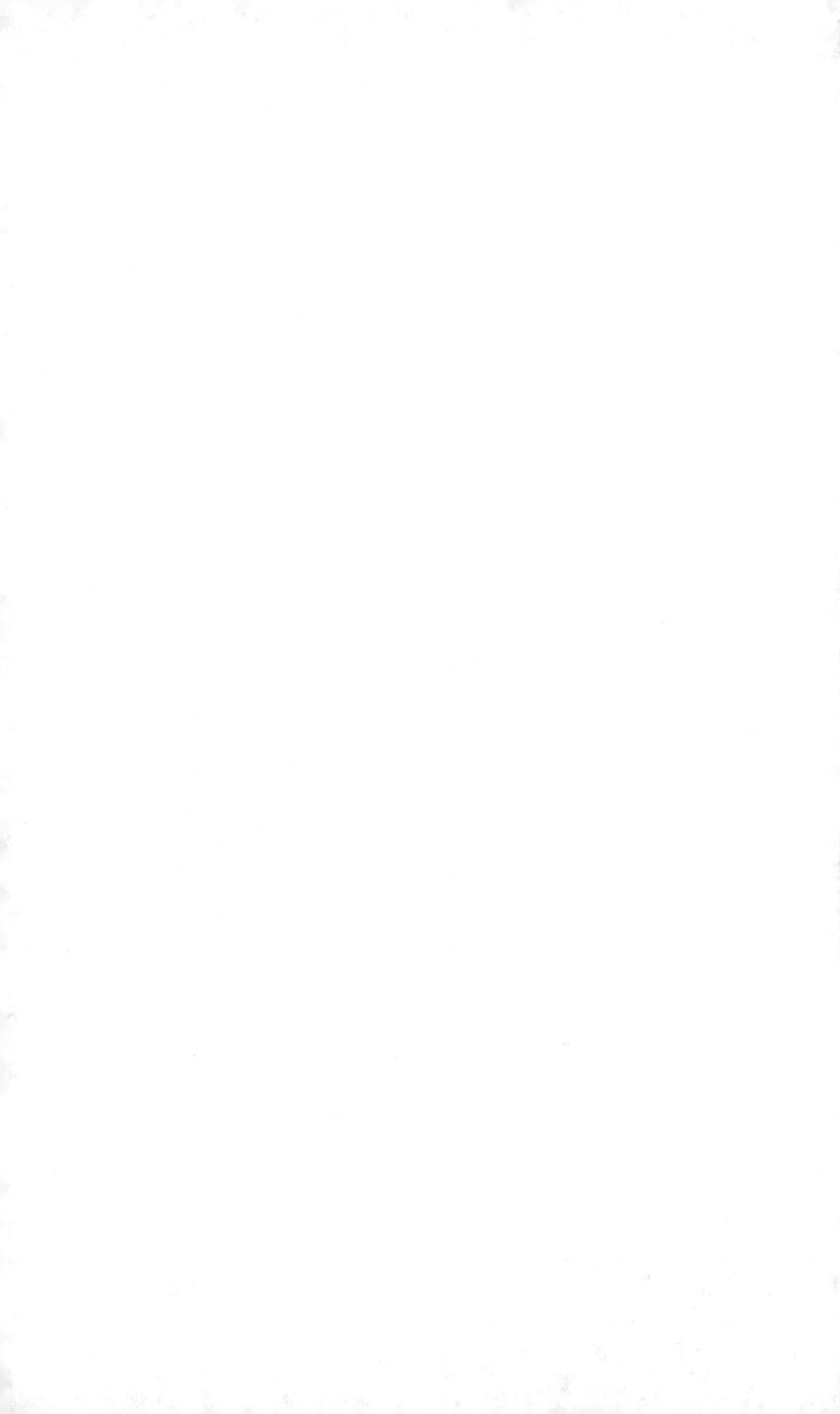